Under Homoeopathy

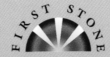

FIRST STONE

Contents

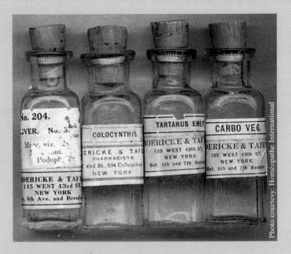

1

Introducing Homoeopathy

Homoeopathy has been an established form of complementary therapy for more than 200 years. It is an 'energy medicine' which stimulates the body's own healing ability.

The essence of homoeopathy is that the whole patient is treated, rather than just the symptoms of illness. Symptoms are seen – quite literally – as expressions of 'dis-ease'. Homoeopathic remedies trigger the body's own healing abilities so that equilibrium is restored to body and mind, and good health results.

Homoeopathy stimulates the body's own healing ability

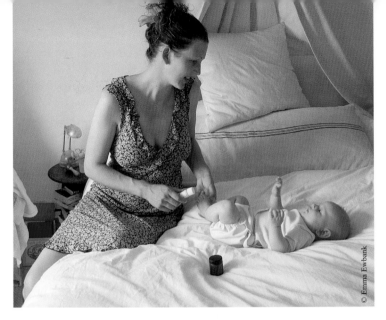

A gentle, non-invasive therapy, homoeopathy can be used on all – from young babies to the elderly.

HOW CAN IT HELP?

As a safe, chemical-free and effective form of medicine, homoeopathy is safe for everyone, from the elderly through to pregnant women and their unborn babies.

Homoeopathy can help nearly all forms of illness. It boosts the immune system, which helps an individual to fight disease. It also raises the general level of health in an individual, improving their overall sense of well-being.

Homoeopathy is often used for diseases that have failed to respond adequately to orthodox medication, such as asthma, eczema, hormonal problems, migraines, and chronic fatigue.

To experience the full benefit of homoeopathy, it is advisable to seek the expertise of an experienced homoeopathic practitioner. However, with guidance, it is also possible for the 'layperson' to self-medicate at home for minor symptoms and for simple first-aid.

2

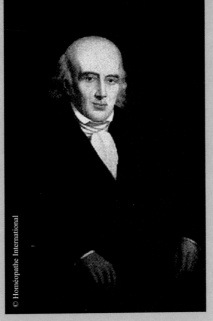

A Brief History

The principles behind homoeopathy date back to the Greek physician Hippocrates in the fifth century BC, and to the Swiss alchemist Paracelsus in the sixteenth century.

Both Hippocrates and Paracelsus were aware of the power of nature to cure disease. Hippocrates realised that there were two ways of treating ill-health: 'the way of opposites' and 'the way of similars'. Conventional medicine tends to rely on the way of opposites, whereas homoeopathy relies on the way of similars.

The name 'homoeopathy' derives from the Greek words 'homoios' (meaning 'similar') and 'pathos' (meaning 'suffering'). It is easy to see how the word 'homoeopathy' became used to describe a medicinal therapy that is based on 'the way of similars'.

HISTORIC USE
Both traditional Chinese medicine and Ayurvedic medicine relate to homoeopathy as they look at

9

the patient holistically, i.e. they believe that, in order to treat the illness, it is necessary to treat the person as a whole.

SAMUEL HAHNEMANN

In 1796, German physician, scholar and chemist Samuel Hahnemann (1755-1843) established the principle *'similia similibus curentur'* which means 'let like be treated by like'. This principle has become a fundamental law of healing, and Hahnemann believed it held the key to curing the sick.

From the time he became a physician in 1779, Hahnemann realised that many methods of orthodox treatment, including blood-letting and administering large doses of chemical agents (such as mercury and arsenic), were far from curative. He also felt it was important to treat every patient, and their disease, as an individual case.

Hahnemann discovered that a substance capable of producing symptoms in a healthy person would cure similar symptoms in a sick person.

PROVINGS

Over a long period of time, Hahnemann and his colleagues took small doses of various substances, some of which were highly poisonous. They wrote down the symptoms produced. These notes were called 'provings'.

Hahnemann's first proving came about after translating a scientific paper on *Cinchona* bark from South America, by Scottish physician William Cullen. The bark produced quinine, which is used in the treatment of malaria. When

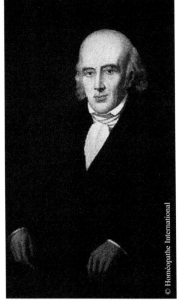

The founder of homoeopathy, Samuel Hahnemann (1755-1843).

© Homéopathe International

11

Hahnemann took the bitter substance himself, he began to experience symptoms similar to those of malaria, with an intermittent fever.

Hahnemann found that, if he stopped taking the *Cinchona*, his symptoms stopped too. He went on to experiment with many people, who all experienced the same symptoms.

After lengthy research into different substances from the animal, vegetable and mineral kingdoms, Hahnemann and his colleagues produced clear results from the substances proved. It was found that patients suffering from similar symptoms to those shown in the provings would experience very positive results if they were treated with the substance used in the proving.

POTENTISATION

After researching provings, Hahnemann developed a system of high dilution, known as 'potentisation'. This not only negated the toxicity of certain substances, but it also heightened the curative

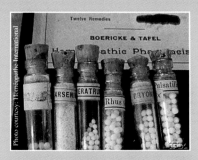

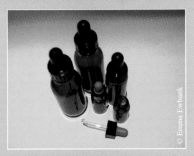

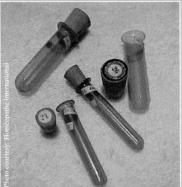

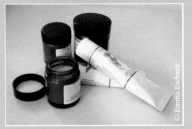

From antique apothecaries to modern medicine. It is surprising how little the tools of the trade have altered, although today's homoeopath can also offer a range of creams and ointments.

powers of the diluted materials. Hahnemann re-tested the potentised *Cinchona* bark on patients suffering with malaria and they improved dramatically.

THE ORGANON

Over the following six years, Hahnemann experimented on himself, his family and his colleagues. His innovative findings were put into a definitive work called the *Organon*. This was completed in 1810, and it is still used today. It remains the ultimate authority on homoeopathy.

LEADING LIGHTS

There were other important figures who contributed to the development of homoeopathy. They include Constantine Hering, Frederick Quin, James Compton Burnett and Edward Bach (a bacteriologist and homoeopath, who created the well-known Bach Flower remedies).

HOMOEOPATHY TODAY

Homoeopathy has, to date, been developed in many countries all over the world. While it has yet to be fully

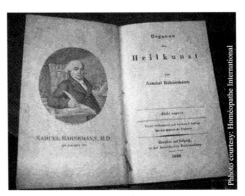

Hahnemann's Organon, first published in 1810, remains the ultimate authority on homoeopathy.

accepted by conventional medicine, its reputation has grown in stature, and it has never been more popular. Indeed, it has been used by several generations of the British royal family.

As a complementary service to traditional medicine, homoeopathy offers an alternative – more natural – approach to health care.

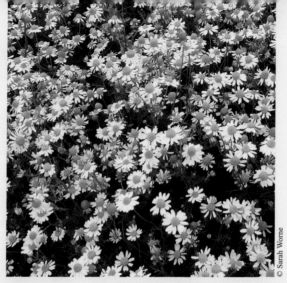
© Sarah Worne

3

How Homoeopathy Works

The mental, emotional and physical symptoms of an illness are different for each individual; no two people are the same.

Homoeopathy differs from conventional medicine because it concentrates on treating the whole patient, not just the disease. A patient's mental and emotional state is considered to be directly related to their physical health.

HEALTH BLOCKS

Health blocks may come in the form of previous (unresolved) disease, past emotional traumas, past physical injuries or vaccination.

Homoeopathy views a person's symptoms as the body's way of overcoming an illness. Homoeopathy aims to stimulate this healing response, not to suppress the body's reaction.

SIMILIA SIMILIBUS CURENTUR (LET LIKE BE TREATED BY LIKE)

In aphorism 26 of his *Organon*, Hahnemann states this law as: "In the living organism, a weaker, dynamic affection is permanently extinguished by a stronger one, which, though different in nature, nevertheless greatly resembles it in expression."

For example, it is well known that contact with raw onions will cause a secretion of tears, with irritation and stinging sensations around the eyes and nose.

Allium cepa is prepared from the common onion, and it is often used for hayfever or colds, which have these similar symptoms.

VITAL FORCE

The human being is a combination of mind, body and spirit, and the vital force is the life energy of each one of us. In acupuncture, it is referred to as 'chi', while in Ayurvedic medicine, the ancient system of medicine in India, the vital force is known as 'prana'. When the vital force is weak or disturbed, we become ill with symptoms of disease.

A homoeopathic remedy is diluted to such an extent that no traceable matter is left.

The potentisation of a remedy (see page 12) releases its energetic nature, which brings about a resonance with our vital force using the Law of Similars (see pages 9 and 17).

A patient receiving a homoeopathic remedy will often notice that they feel better 'in themselves' some time before their physical symptoms improve. This is because a homoeopathic remedy works by restoring the body's vital force, which has the effect of increasing a person's energy levels.

LAW AND DIRECTION OF CURE

Constantine Hering (1800-1880), the father of American homoeopathy, observed a process known as Hering's Law of Cure.

This principle states that, during the process of disease and healing, a person's symptoms will appear in one order and disappear in the reverse order. Homoeopathic patients may also experience symptoms during their healing process that they may have contracted in the past.

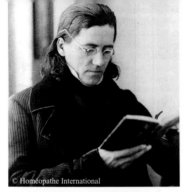
Constantine Hering – the father of American homoeopathy.

Another homoeopathic principle is that, as a disease progresses, it will move from the periphery to the centre. Therefore, healing needs to work from the inside out.

REMEDIES
Homoeopathic remedies are made from plant, animal and mineral properties. Many of these substances are poisonous to humans in large material doses, such as snake and spider venom, deadly nightshade, and the minerals mercury and arsenic.

Plants are usually soaked in a mixture of alcohol and water to make a 'mother tincture', which is then potentised by a series of dilutions and succussions. Succussion is a method of shaking the remedy in order to enhance it further.

Other substances, such as pure flint (*Silica*) or silver (*Arg. nit.*), are triturated (ground up) with lactose or milk sugar before they are further diluted by potentisation (see page 12).

DILUTION

There are two main methods of dilution – decimal and centesimal.

The ratio of 1:10 (decimal) is denoted by an x or d and 1:100 (centesimal) is denoted by a c.

POTENCY

Homoeopathic remedies come in a range of potencies. To determine the strength of a remedy, look at the number – the higher the number, the more powerful the remedy.

Potencies 6x, 6c and 30c are commonly sold over the counter. Higher potencies, such as 200c, 1m (one in a thousand), 10m (one in 10 thousand) and cm (one hundred thousand), are best prescribed by a practitioner. They are not advised for use at home.

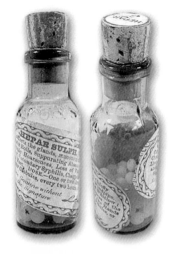

4

The Benefits Of Homoeopathy

There are many benefits of using homoeopathy, which make this established system of medicine an important and valuable choice for maintaining good health in today's world.

The main benefits of homoeopathy are that:

- It is an holistic medicine
- It is safe for everyone
- It encourages personal growth
- It is affordable
- It does not involve animal-testing.

HOLISTIC MEDICINE

Holistic medicine takes a wider view of illness and treats each person as an individual. With the pace of life speeding up, the level of daily stress also increases. It is important to keep our lives in balance if we are to remain healthy. With its holistic approach, homoeopathy is ideally suited to the task of keeping a person's life in balance.

Homoeopaths record each patient's case thoroughly and comprehensively, taking factors such as lifestyle habits very seriously.

During the initial consultation, the homoeopath will spend considerable time with the patient to establish where that person may be overextending themselves or holding back in life, be it physically or emotionally.

Although the consultation is a very important part of the process, it is the remedy that holds the key. It engages with the patient's own vital force, which initiates the body's healing powers.

Babies and animals are excellent examples of how remedies work effectively, and, because they cannot talk to the practitioner, it shows that homoeopathic remedies are not placebos (a sense of benefit felt by a patient that arises solely from the knowledge that treatment has been given).

SAFE FOR EVERYONE
It is possible for everyone to benefit from homoeopathy, from unborn babies to the elderly and infirm. The

remedies have no danger of poisoning, nor can they cause any damage.

The fact that remedies are so diluted takes away the danger of overdosing, and there are no harmful side effects. There may be a slight reaction of sorts, but this is temporary and part of the body's healing process to rid itself of disease.

Homoeopathy is effective in emergency situations where there is shock, severe bleeding, serious physical injury and head injuries.

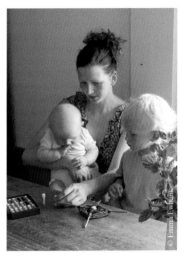

One of the main benefits of homoeopathy is that it is safe for babies and toddlers.

25

Serious injuries always need expert treatment, but you can use remedies to help you while you are on the way to the hospital. For example, *Arnica* can be used to treat shock and injury.

Extreme emotional shock, such as bereavement, can also be helped enormously with homoeopathy.

PERSONAL GROWTH

Homoeopathy is essentially about increasing a person's energy. This automatically increases a patient's sense of well-being, which, in turn, strengthens the will to deal with any stress that may be part of his or her life.

An increase in energy brings about an increase in confidence, helping individuals move forward to lead more fulfilled lives. It gives them the strength to make any necessary changes.

Depression and anxiety hold back our personal development and stop us from living life to the full. Homoeopathy can help enormously with these mental and emotional states that have become out of balance.

Homoeopathy also has the potential to move people forward in their spiritual lives. As a patient evolves, they are able to find their right path in life. As this happens, they begin to experience, and get in touch with, their inner self, and feel a greater sense of peace.

Homoeopathy is an effective tool that has the power to change our consciousness so we can achieve a better and more enriched life.

AFFORDABLE

Homoeopathic remedies are usually less costly than other forms of medication. A homoeopathic consultation may appear to be an expensive outlay initially, but in contrast to its benefits in long-term health, it is relatively inexpensive. You will not need to visit your homoeopath as frequently, and, as your health improves, the period between appointments will lengthen.

Homoeopathic remedies are also less expensive to produce than orthodox medication.

Homoeopathy not only deals with a person's immediate complaints but it also changes his/her overall susceptibility to disease – for the better. This raises a person's general level of health for themselves and for future generations.

Using homoeopathy as a preventative method of treatment is a good form of insurance, laying down an excellent foundation for health.

NO ANIMAL-TESTING

Homoeopathic remedies are tested on human beings, not on animals.

Today, the 'proving' of a remedy is organised by a group of volunteers, who, under supervision, are given a homoeopathic dose of a substance over a period of time. These are healthy individuals, who, in time, will produce a range of symptoms from the remedy taken. These symptoms are then recorded.

The collective experience is the basis for understanding the 'picture' of the remedy. All the information is used, according to the Law of Similars (see pages 9 and 10), to prescribe for a patient with the same symptoms.

There are hundreds of established homoeopathic remedies, and new remedies are consistently being proved to respond to our ever changing world (see Chapter Seven).

A FURTHER BENEFIT
Homoeopathy is excellent for keeping babies and children healthy, especially for parents who do not wish to vaccinate their children. In such situations, it is vital to maintain children in good health; a good diet is not sufficient.

Homoeopathy is also an effective method to bring a child back into balance after vaccination, especially if parents notice a change in their child's vitality. This applies to adults too, if they have also never felt well since an inoculation.

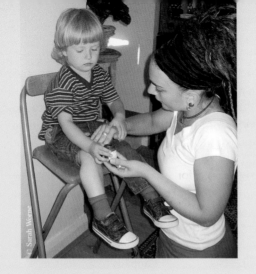

5 Will Homoeopathy Work For Me?

Homoeopathy is suitable for all people and nearly every situation. The following uses are just some examples.

FIRST-AID

Homoeopathy can be used for any injury and accident. If you have a serious injury, you may need orthodox treatment (for example, to treat a broken bone), but there are many remedies that can be used before and after the setting of a bone to speed up recovery.

Homoeopathy is also of great value to any sporting injury. *Arnica* (see page 50) is homoeopathy's number one first-aid remedy and no one should be without it.

TRAVEL

Homoeopathic remedies are easy and compact to take away on a holiday and for extensive travelling.

A homoeopathic first-aid kit is a wise investment and takes up no space at all!

Homoeopathic remedies can be used for sunburn, stomach upsets, travel sickness, fevers

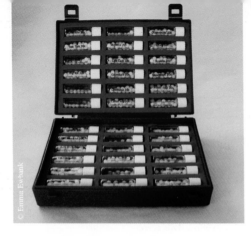

A homoeopathic first-aid kit is a wise investment for travellers.

and jet-lag. They are simple and easy to take – a bonus for any traveller.

MINOR AILMENTS

Many common complaints can be treated successfully with homoeopathy.

One of the main advantages of homoeopathic remedies is that it reduces the need to take strong medication as well

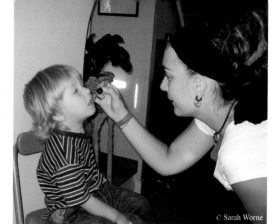

Children usually love taking homoeopathic remedies.

© Sarah Worne

as helping to alleviate discomfort.

CHILDREN
Homoeopathy is an ideal system of medicine for babies and children, who are often prone to fevers, painful teething, earaches, colds and coughs. They taste pleasant and most children love taking them!

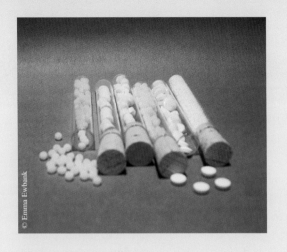
© Emma Ewbank

6 Using Homoeopathy

Taking homoeopathic remedies is very simple: they should be put straight into a clean mouth, without water, and sucked for a few minutes.

Some people put them under their tongue. Powders and liquid remedies can be dropped into the mouth, straight on to the tongue.

CAUTION

The curing power of remedies can be antidoted, and it is important not to touch the remedies with your hands –

especially if you are giving a remedy to someone else.

Keep the homoeopathic remedies away from electrical and magnetic devices, especially mobile telephones, strong odours, heat and direct sunlight.

Make sure you do not eat or drink approximately 10 minutes before or after taking a remedy to give it the best possible chance of working effectively.

It is advisable to cut out stimulating drinks, such as coffee and strong tea; while undergoing homoeopathic treatment. This is because these drinks can disturb the curative response – or even antidote – the remedy that you are taking.

Strong-smelling substances can also antidote remedies. Strong aromatic oils (such as tea-tree oil, camphor and menthol), and scented products (including toothpaste, mints, throat lozenges, some cough mixtures and vapour rubs/inhalations) should be avoided.

CONVENTIONAL MEDICATION

There are a number of medications and procedures that can affect the power of homoeopathic remedies. These include:

- Immunisations, including flu and tetanus vaccines and holiday jabs.
- Hormone-based medication, such as the contraceptive pill and hormone replacement therapy.
- Dental treatment.
- X-rays.

If you have a concern about mixing prescribed orthodox medication with homoeopathy, it is important to discuss the matter with your doctor and homoeopath. Do not stop taking your medication because you think it may affect your remedies – always check first.

During the initial consultation with your homoeopath, you will be asked to provide details of any medication you are taking or any medical procedures you have had or are about to receive. It is very important that you supply this information as thoroughly as possible.

TREATING SPECIFIC PROBLEMS

Homoeopathy can be effective for all conditions, but it is important to seek the advice of a professional if there are long-standing symptoms or symptoms that are not responding to self-treatment. Repeated bouts of symptoms may indicate an underlying condition that requires the expertise of an experienced practitioner.

There are two types of symptoms – acute and chronic.

ACUTE ILLNESSES
These include:
- Common colds, coughs, sore throats, etc.
- Nausea
- Minor gastric problems, such as mild diarrhoea and indigestion

If your symptoms continue, or if they improve to begin with only to return later, your body is expressing an underlying chronic condition that requires expert treatment. If this happens, your body is trying to tell you something!

CHRONIC ILLNESSES
Chronic diseases are those that exist for a long time or that appear again and again. They include:
- Asthma
- Arthritis
- Migraine
- Skin diseases
- Allergies.

Chronic conditions should be

treated only under the supervision of a professional and experienced homoeopath.

Some chronic conditions that can respond particularly well to homoeopathic remedies include:

- Migraines
- Insomnia
- PMT
- Menopause
- Asthma
- Eczema
- Vertigo
- Chronic fatigue
- Digestive disorders
- Depression.

WHEN TO CONSULT A PROFESSIONAL

Generally speaking, it is always wise to consult a professional homoeopath when you first start using homoeopathy. However, if you choose to self-prescribe, there are certain situations when you will still need to see a professional:

- When self-prescribing is not working
- When acute illness keeps repeating itself
- If you feel out of balance mentally and emotionally, e.g. stress

- After an acute illness, such as influenza, to re-balance your immune system
- If you have a range of minor complaints
- To maintain a good level of health.

A HOMOEOPATHIC CONSULTATION

The initial consultation can take anything from between one and two hours, depending on the individual homoeopath. A full history needs to be recorded, covering your medical history, mental, emotional and physical make-up, and inherited family history.

Significant physical and emotional traumas are important, and you will be asked to describe your symptoms in your own words.

All this information is gathered together by the homoeopath to work out your general constitution and to ascertain what 'blocks' (see page 17) need to be removed to aid your cure and to allow you to contine in good health.

WHAT HAPPENS NEXT?

Many patients experience a sense of well-being, often before their physical ailments disappear. Once a good level of health has been maintained, however, it is important to continue to visit your homoeopath to keep your level of health constant.

Your case and current lifestyle will be re-assessed and the appropriate remedy will be given to increase your energy and to keep you in balance, supporting your immune system. Stress lowers our immune system significantly, making us more susceptible to disease, which is why homoeopaths strive to keep the body in balance – prevention is better than cure!

FAMILY LINKS

Homoeopathy is ideal for babies and children to ensure good health. It can significantly lessen the need for medication, such as antibiotics or steroids.

Homoeopathy also has the potential to help overcome hereditary disease. The illnesses in our family line can sometimes weaken various aspects of our own health. That is why it is important for a homoeopath to take down a full family history and connect any patterns of illness causing possible areas of weakness within the patient.

If you are receiving professional homoeopathic treatment and physical symptoms arise (an acute illness), do not try to treat yourself before you have consulted your homoeopath. Your symptoms may well be part of your cure, and a necessary process that should not be interfered with. This is considered a 'cleansing' process, which is a good sign and shows that treatment is progressing in the right direction. Rest and a refined, cleansing diet may be all that you need to work through these temporary symptoms.

APPOINTMENTS

Appointment frequency can vary from between three weeks and three months, depending on your general level of health, and your homoeopath's regime.

LEARNING MORE

For anyone new to homoeopathy, it is advisable to first seek the help of an experienced homoeopathic practitioner.

Should you wish to learn more, there are many books on homoeopathy for beginners. You may also choose to benefit from taking a homoeopathic first-aid course, to give you more confidence in self-prescribing.

Your local homoeopath may run courses, and local education authorities often run part-time courses for you to learn more. Practical application is a good way to learn how the remedies work.

Health shops are good sources of information to find a local homoeopath. Alternatively, contact The Society of Homeopaths, which will advise you how to find your nearest registered practitioner who has undergone approved formal training (see page 61).

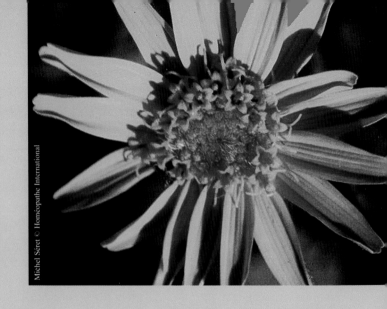

Michel Séret © Homéopathe International

7

Remedy Selection

There is a vast number of homoeopathic remedies. They can be used for minor and/or acute illness and first-aid situations.

If you are going to self-prescribe, you will need to be familiar with common symptoms and learn to observe them, however subtle they may be.

If symptoms persist, it is always important to seek professional advice.

For serious accidents and emergencies, homoeopathic first-aid can help a tremendous amount for shock and trauma while you are on your way to hospital.

SELF-PRESCRIBING

If the retailer from whom you purchase your remedies does not supply remedy information, it is advisable to purchase a simple book on homoeopathy. This should inform you about basic symptoms and how to select the correct remedy. Various books will provide you with information on how to

45

compile your own homoeopathic first-aid kit – ideal for use at home or to take travelling.

Practical application is the only way to gain experience and to increase your confidence in self-prescribing.

SYMPTOMS

In order to choose the best homoeopathic remedy, it is important to note symptoms and to take into account the following:

- How did the symptom start? Suddenly or slowly?
- Was there a trigger of any kind (physical or emotional)?
- Take the emotional picture into account. How are you feeling – happy, sad, angry or clingy?
- Where is the location of the symptom? Ear, nose, throat, stomach, etc.?
- What is the sensation/quality of discomfort? For example, sharp, dull, throbbing, needle-like, bruised?
- What makes you feel better or worse? Heat, cold, fresh air, time of day, position?
- What is the temperature?

Do you feel hot or cold, on the inside or the outside? What about your extremities (fingers, toes, etc.)?

- Changes in appetite and thirst. Is there any particular food or drink that is preferred? What about the quantity?
- Is there any kind of discharge? If so, what is the colour and odour? Is it irritating or bland?

SELECTING A REMEDY

Once you have noted your symptoms, you need to find a remedy that has as close a fit to those symptoms as possible.

You may find there are several remedies with the same physical symptoms. Choose two or three of the closest and then make your selection from the nearest mental and emotional symptoms.

If you have given six doses of a remedy with no signs of improvement, this is an indication to move on to another appropriate remedy with a similar symptom picture.

It is important to use one remedy only at a time. If your chosen remedy doesn't have the desired effect, move on to another one. Remember, if symptoms persist, it is essential to seek professional advice. Always get medical attention when urgently needed.

DOSAGE

The main principle is: 'use the minimum dose'. Give a remedy for the amount of time it takes to initiate a healing response. Therefore, it is important to stop giving the remedy once the symptoms have improved.

Timing will depend on the severity of the symptom. If there is a sudden onset, accompanied by severe pain, give remedies more frequently. For example, in a first-aid situation, such as a fall (which usually results in bruising and swelling to a limb), *Arnica*, given every 30 minutes, would be the first remedy to think of. Stop on improvement, and repeat as needed if pain or discomfort return.

Less immediate physical symptoms, such as colds, flu

and children's teething, can be dosed every four hours or three to four times a day.

As symptoms improve, the dose can be given less frequently. Stop the remedy altogether when symptoms cease.

REMEDY POTENCY
Remedies come in a variety of strengths (see page 21). For basic self-prescribing, the lower potencies are more appropriate, such as 6c and 30c, which can be bought at most good chemists.

As a general rule, for 6c potencies, take one pill three to six times a day until symptoms improve.

For 30c potencies, take one pill up to one to three times a day until symptoms improve.

REMEDY CHOICES
Homoeopathic pharmacies will be able to offer a selection of remedies. There are hard tablets, ball-shaped pillules, poppyseed-sized granules (suitable for babies), and soft, melt-in-the-mouth pills (which are ideal for small children,

and, when crushed, for babies as well).

Remedies can also be bought in liquid form (in an alcohol dilution), or as individual, single powders.

Homoeopathic remedies are available in sugar-free and lactose-free varieties for those with extreme sugar and dairy intolerances.

BASIC HOMOEOPATHIC FIRST-AID REMEDIES

The following remedies are to be used in 6c or 30c potency. Give one dose and wait to see what relief it brings. Repeat the dose according to the urgency of the situation – three to four hours on average – stepping up to every 30 minutes for very acute symptoms.

If in doubt, it is best to contact your homoeopath; in an emergency, seek expert medical attention or go straight to hospital.

ARNICA
- **Proper name:** *Arnica montana*
- **Common name:** Mountain Daisy

Arnica is found all over the world, growing on the slopes of mountain valleys. It is suitable for all trauma – mental and physical – whether recent or in the past. It is the number one remedy for accident injuries, shock, and physical exhaustion. It helps to speed up recovery and reduce any soreness or bruising.

Arnica is especially good for operations. It helps the body to cope with the invasiveness and shock of surgery, which, in turn, helps to reduce

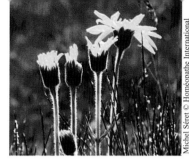

Arnica should be the first choice of remedy for treating accident injuries and shock.

Michel Séret © Homéopathe International

soreness and speed up recovery. It is also a beneficial treatment for those recovering from dental treatment and for women who have just given birth.

Arnica is an essential remedy for any sportsperson who needs an injury dealt with promptly, to avoid loss of play. A bottle of *Arnica* can be kept in a kit bag for use as soon as injury occurs.

Arnica is not just for the sportsperson, however. It is great for bruising, sprains and strains caused by overexertion – even too much gardening or housework! It will also help a great deal with relieving weariness and aching muscles after a sleepless night.

Arnica is an essential remedy to keep at home, in the car, or, better still, carried with you.

Arnica can be used externally as a cream, but it should never be applied to broken skin.

Once you have experienced the healing power of *Arnica* on a bruised muscle or sprain, you will never want to be without it again.

ACONITE
- **Proper name:** *Aconite napellus*
- **Common name:** Monkshood

Aconite is excellent for shock and fear, and it is also useful for the early stages of colds and fevers. It needs to be given at the onset, when symptoms come on suddenly, especially after exposure to windy weather.

APIS
- **Proper name:** *Apis mellifica*
- **Common name:** Honey Bee

Apis is an excellent choice for the treatment of bites, stings and hives. It is also suitable for

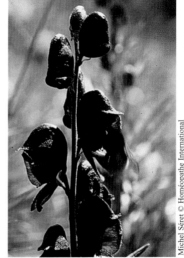

Aconite *can be used to help prevent severe symptoms of colds and fevers.*

Michel Séret © Homéopathe International

53

general inflammation, where the skin is red, and for allergic reactions. *Urtica urens* (stinging nettle) is another good remedy for skin irritation.

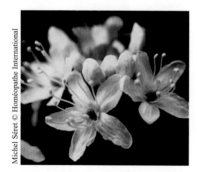

Michel Séret © Homéopathe International

Use Ledum for bites, puncture wounds and black eyes.

LEDUM
- **Proper name:** *Ledum palustre*
- **Common name:** Marsh Tea

Ledum contains anti-tetanus properties and helps to fight infection. It is a specific remedy for puncture wounds and bites, and an excellent treatment for black eyes.

HYPERICUM
- **Proper name:** *Hypericum perforatum*
- **Common name:** St. John's Wort

The versatility of St. John's Wort has long been established. The potentised homoeopathic form of *Hypericum* is very good for the treatment of injuries to nerve-rich areas, such as fingers and toes. It is also effective for lacerated wounds and shooting nerve pain. It contains anti-tetanus properties, similar to ledum.

CALENDULA

- **Proper name:** *Calendula officinalis*
- **Common name:** Marigold

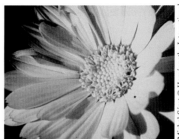

Calendula *is derived from the marigold, and is great for wounds and superficial burns.*

Use *Calendula* to aid the healing of wounds and superficial burns. *Cantharis* (Spanish fly) is another suitable choice of remedy for burns.

Calendula can be used

55

externally as a cream or diluted tincture, but make sure the wound is clean before application. Used internally, *Calendula* can help to fight infection after an operation.

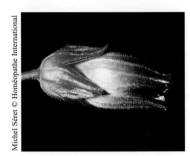

Michel Séret © Homéopathe International

Belladonna – *a blessing for those suffering from severe fever.*

BELLADONNA
- **Proper name:** *Atropa belladonna*
- **Common name:** Deadly Nightshade

Belladonna is extremely useful for the treatment of high fevers, particularly those with a sudden onset. It can be used to treat a specific inflamed area or when the patient's body is burning, red and hot.

Belladonna is an appropriate remedy for violent, throbbing pains and sunstroke.

CHAMOMILLA

- **Proper name:** *Matricaria chamomilla*
- **Common name:** Chamomile

The parents of teething children should never be without *Chamomilla*. It is excellent for controlling severe pain. Adults can also use it to soothe toothache.

Chamomilla is also very good to give to bad-tempered children who quieten when carried and who constantly request then reject things.

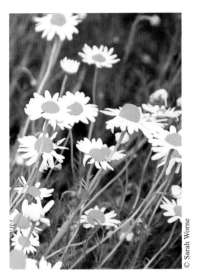

© Sarah Worne

Use Chamomilla *to control toothache and bad-tempered children!*

ARSENICUM
- **Proper name:** *Arsenicum album*
- **Common name:** Arsenic Trioxide

Use *Arsenicum* for food poisoning, when the patient shows signs of anxiousness, restlessness and thirst. Other common symptoms include burning pains and a desire for warmth and warm/hot drinks.

PULSATILLA
- **Proper name:** *Pulsatilla pratensis*
- **Common name:** Wind Flower

Pulsatilla is an effective remedy for the emotionally tearful and those who crave company. In particular, it can

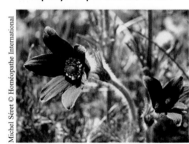

Michel Séret © Homéopathe International

Pulsatilla *can be used to soothe whining children.*

be given to children who whinge or are clingy.

Common symptoms indicating this remedy include a lack of thirst and signs of improvement when the patient is out in fresh air. Ear infections with similar emotional symptoms can also be treated with *Pulsatilla,* as can head colds and catarrh (yellow, thick, bland mucous).

Pulsatilla can also help relieve the effects of overindulgence of fatty foods (e.g. pork or pastries). *Nux vomica* (Poison Nut) is an alternative remedy for overindulgence, especially alcohol-induced ones (hangovers)!

HYPERCAL TINCTURE
This is a combination of *Calendula* and *Hypericum.*

Hypercal tincture is used externally. It can be applied to superficial skin injuries to stimulate healing. It needs to be diluted – one teaspoon to a pint of clean water or 10-20 drops to one tumbler-full.

FURTHER REMEDIES
Homoeopathic creams can be

bought over the counter from most good chemists. They make a great addition to your homoeopathic first-aid kit. They include *Arnica, Calendula, Hypericum, Rhus tox* and *Ruta*.

Homoeopathic creams are ideal for babies and toddlers, especially when treating nappy rash, as they all have excellent therapeutic qualities but are very mild and gentle.

Please note that, in cases of eczema, it is important to use a cream that allows the skin to breathe. While the healing properties of *Calendula* are gentle, it is not ideal for eczema cases, as it is capable of sealing the skin. If in doubt, contact a qualified homoeopath.

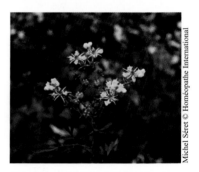

Ruta – *a useful remedy to keep in your first-aid kit.*

How To Find Us

In the UK, there are five homoeopathic hospitals and homoeopathy is practised all over the world. An internet search will reveal the main governing body in each country.

ORGANISATIONS
The Society of Homeopaths,
11 Brookfield Duncan Close,
Moulton Park,
Northampton,
NN3 6WL.
Tel: 0845 450 6611
Fax: 0845 450 6622
Email: info@homeopathy.soh.org
Website: www.homeopathy-soh.org

British Homeopathic Association,
Hahnemann House,
29 Park Street West,
Luton, LU1 3BE.
Tel: 0870 444 3950
Website: www.trusthomeopathy.org

The following websites may be useful for anyone looking for homoeopathic remedies:
www.helioslondon.com
www.helios.co.uk
www.ainsworths.com
A. Nelson and Co. Ltd. and Weleda also make homoeopathic remedies that can be found in most large chemists and health-food stores.

About the author

Sarah Worne graduated from the London College of Practical Homoeopathy in 1995, and she is a registered member of The Society of Homeopaths. Sarah manages her own clinic at the Lewes Subud Centre in Lewes, East Sussex, as well as working at The Integrated Medical Centre, New Cavendish Street, London. She also runs homoeopathic workshops, including first-aid courses.

For further information, please contact Sarah on:
www.leweshomoeopathy.com
sjworne@leweshomoeopathy.com

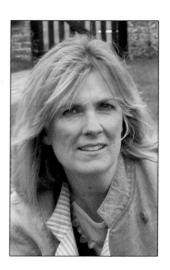

Other titles in the series

- **Understanding Acupressure**
- **Understanding Acupuncture**
- **Understanding The Alexander Technique**
- **Understanding Aloe Vera**
- **Understanding Bach Flower Remedies**
- **Understanding The Bowen Technique**
- **Understanding Craniosacral Therapy**
- **Understanding Echinacea**
- **Understanding Fish Oils**
- **Understanding Garlic**
- **Understanding Indian Head Massage**
- **Understanding Kinesiology**
- **Understanding Massage**
- **Understanding Reiki**
- **Understanding St. John's Wort**
- **Understanding Shiatsu**
- **Understanding Yoga**

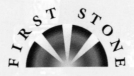

First published 2005 by First Stone Publishing
PO Box 8, Lydney, Gloucestershire, GL15 6YD

The contents of this book are for information only and are not intended as a substitute for appropriate medical attention. The author and publishers admit no liability for any consequences arising from following any advice contained within this book. If you have any concerns about your health or medication, always consult your doctor.

Cover photography: Main image © Emma Ewbank;
Sub image Michel Serét © Homéopathe International.
All other photography © as stated

ISBN 1 904439 40 3

Printed and bound in Hong Kong through Printworks International Ltd.